Harmony's™ House
... a storybook to color

WRITTEN BY
Margery Phelps and David Allen, Pd.D.

ILLUSTRATIONS BY
Michael Carney and Tanya Pash

ISBN-13: 978-1508738596

ISBN-10: 1508738599

a publication of

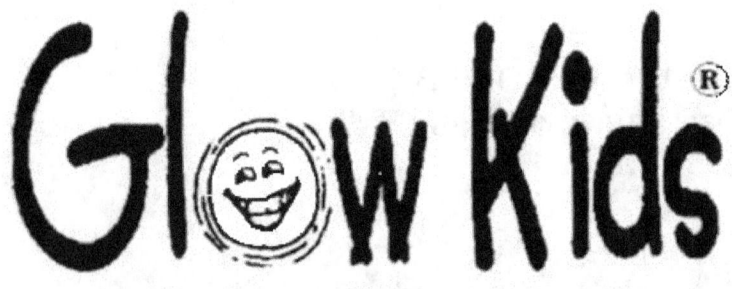

leading the children of the world to wellness

www.GlowKids.net

This is Harmony, the healthy cell

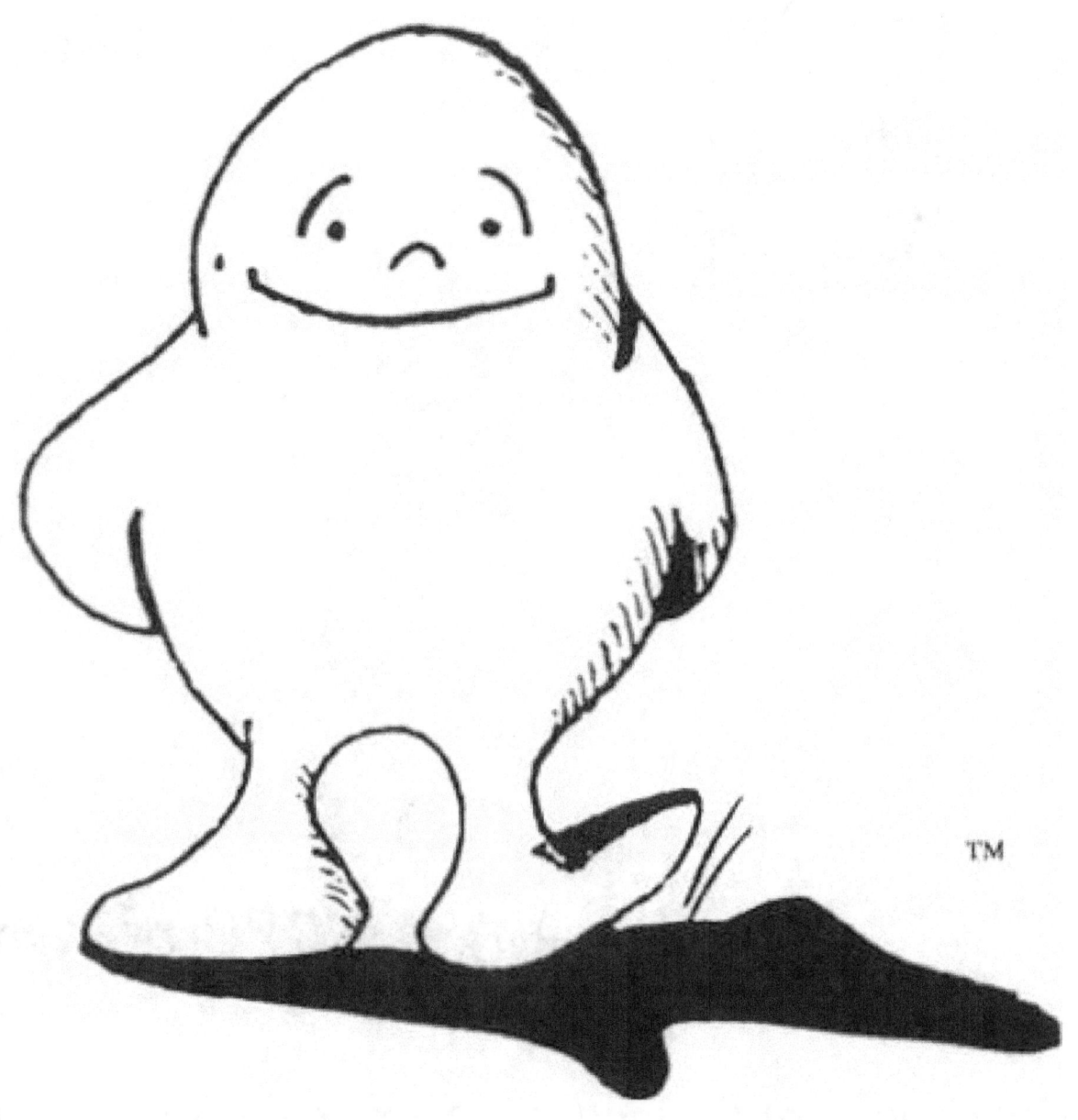

You have 75,000,000,000,000

cells in your precious body.

Your body is your home.

It's the most important home you will ever have.

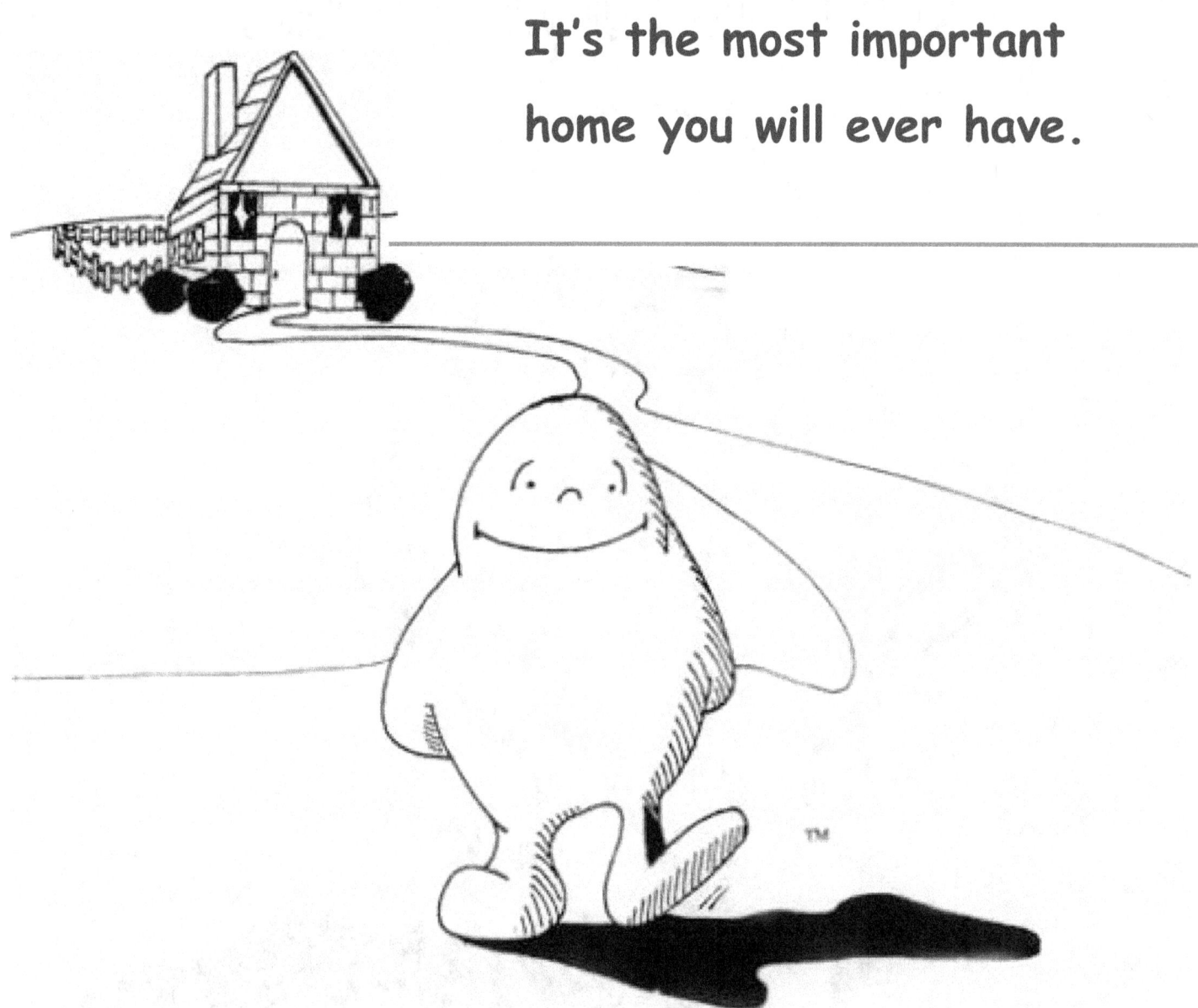

When you take good care of your home, you will be healthy – and Harmony will be happy!

If your body is your Home, your mouth is the front door.

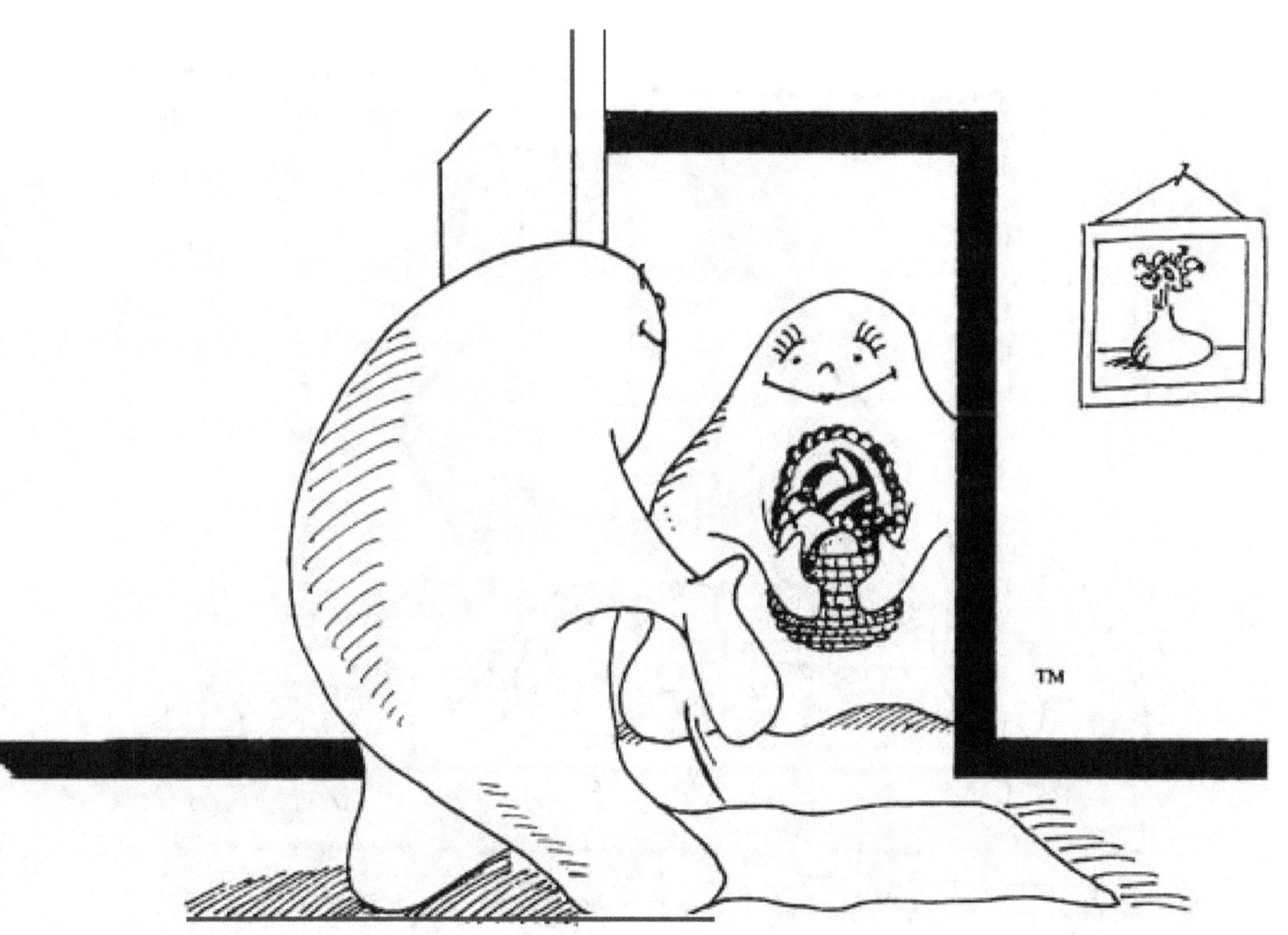

What do you invite into your home?

Fruits and Vegetables are good for your Home.

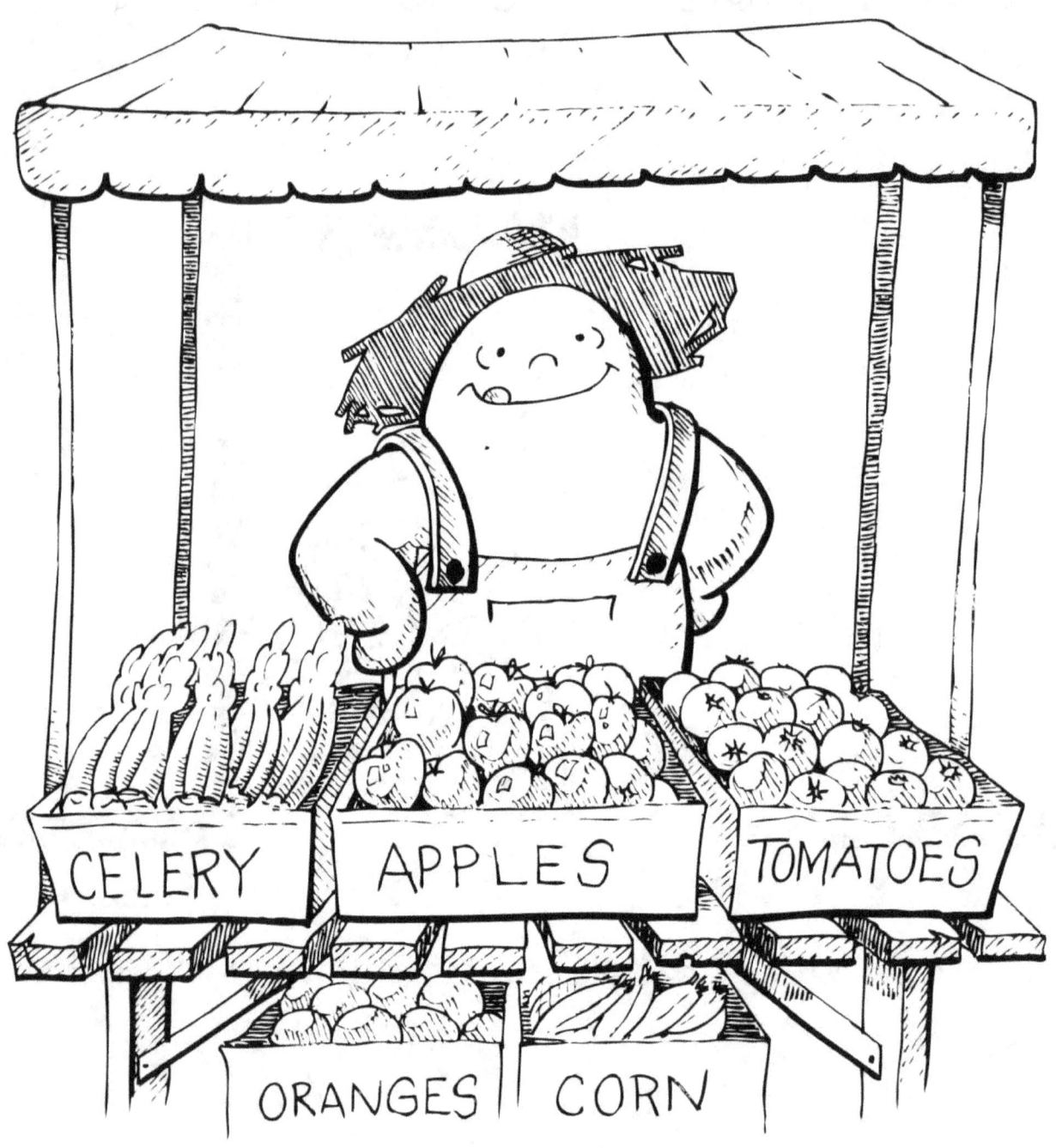

CELERY   APPLES   TOMATOES

ORANGES   CORN

When Harmony has lots of these, you'll feel great!

Uh, oh. What happened to Harmony?

You need to drink plenty of water
to keep Harmony clean.

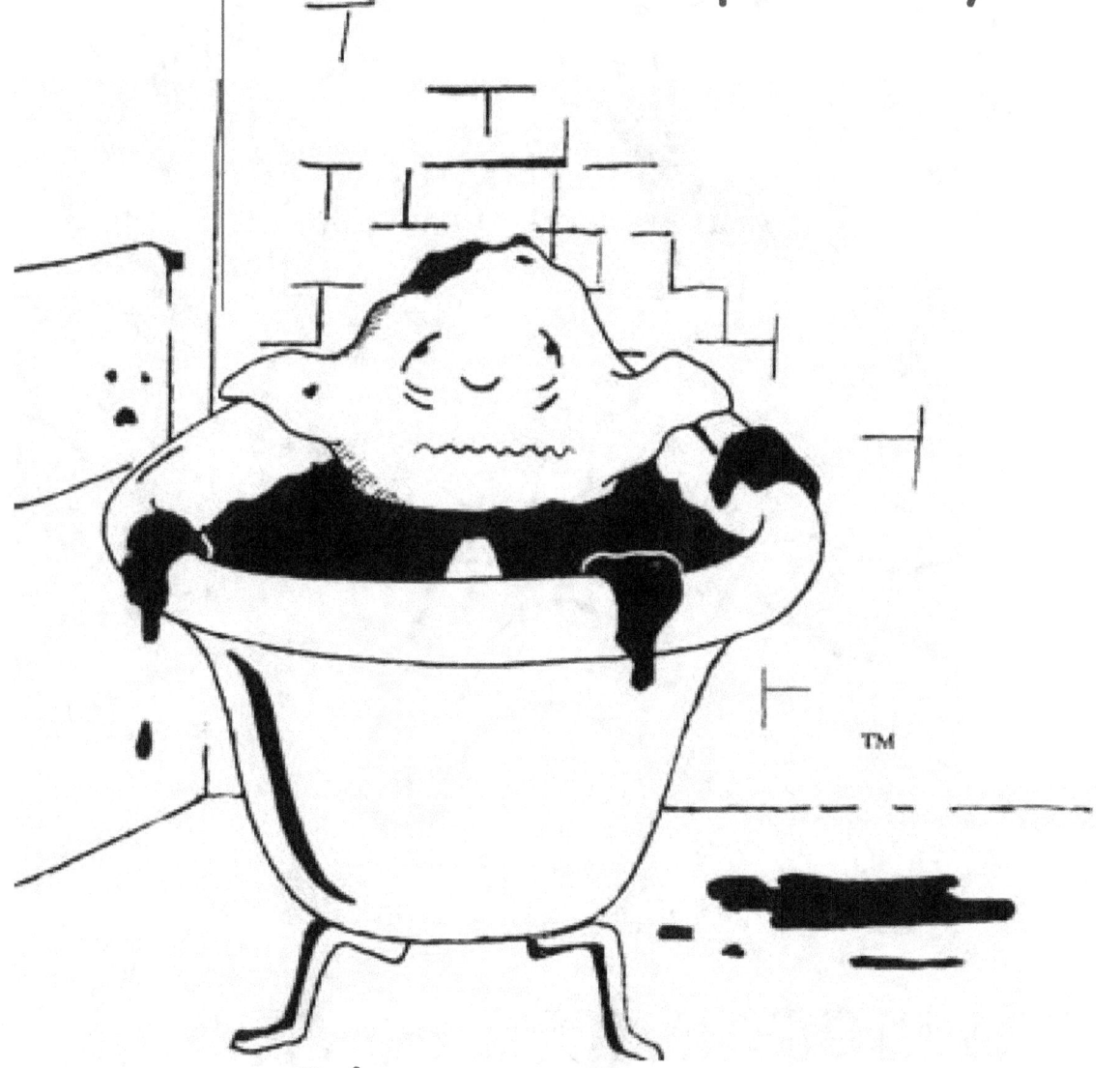

Colas are not water.

They make a mess in your home.

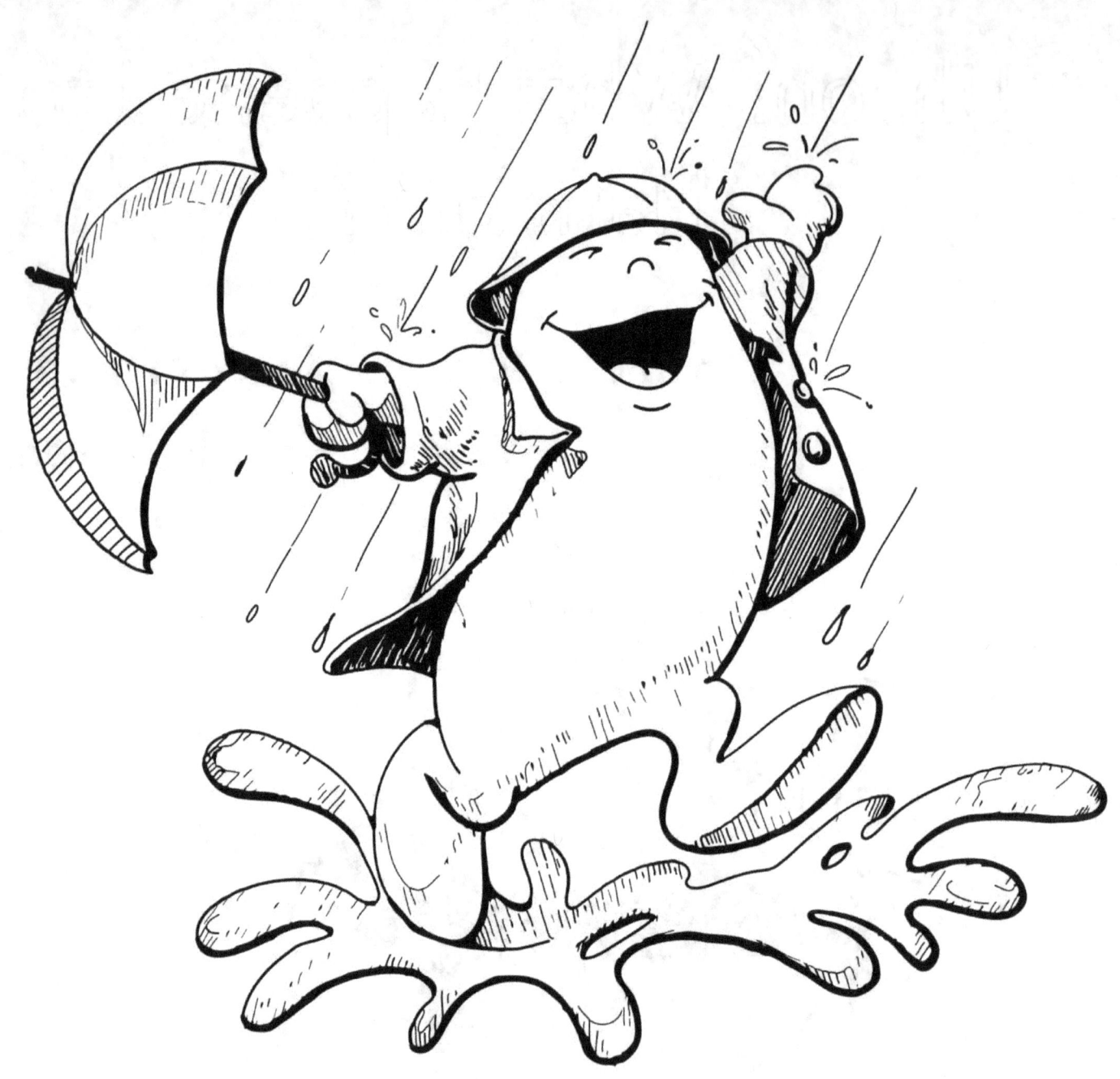

So, be sure you

shower Harmony
with clean water every day...

...that means you drink lots of water!

If your body is your Home, your stomach is the Kitchen,

the place where food is prepared.

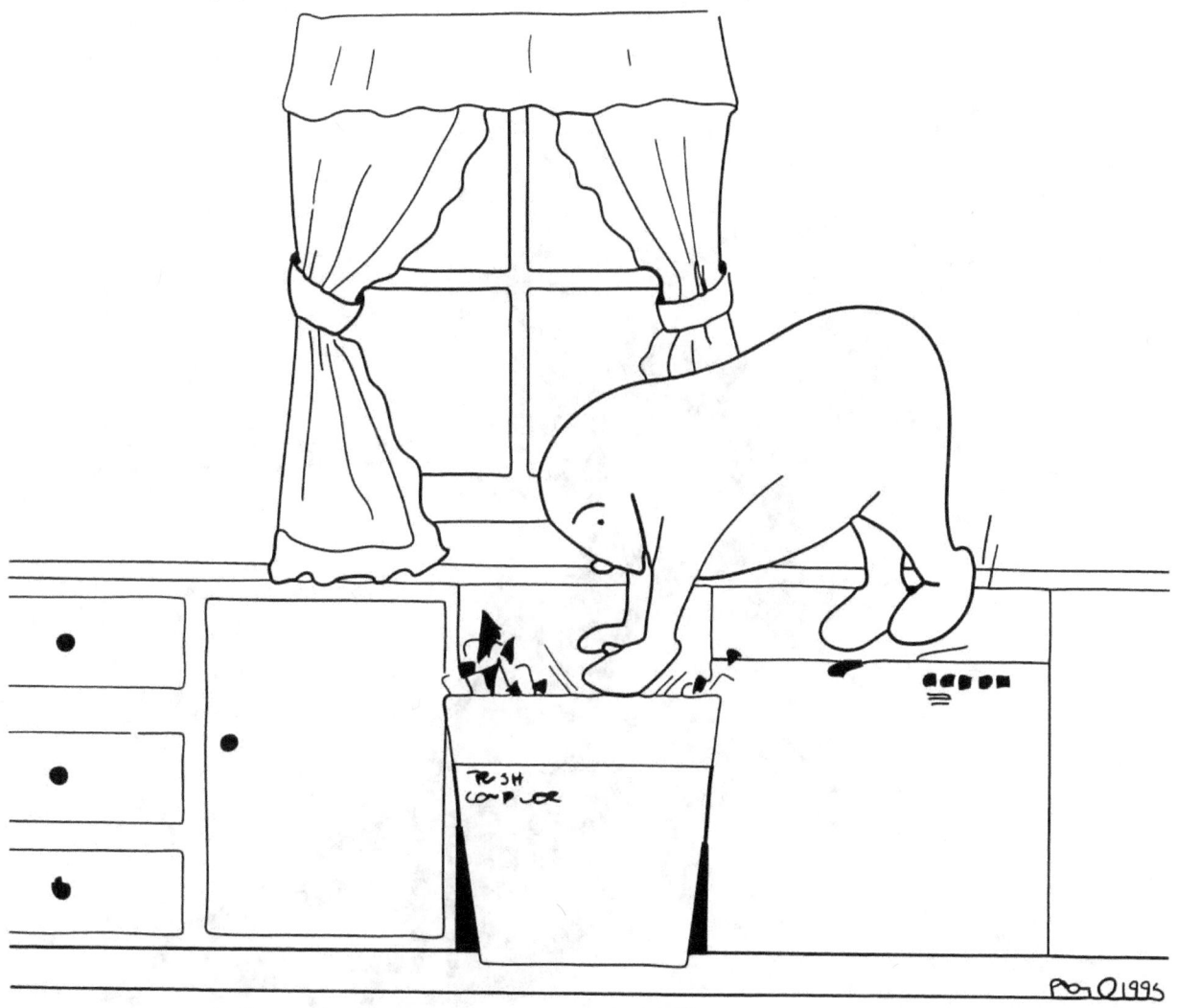

After you eat, you need to clean up the kitchen. In Harmony's house that means you should go to the bathroom regularly to get rid of waste.

Harmony needs fuel to keep the furnace running.

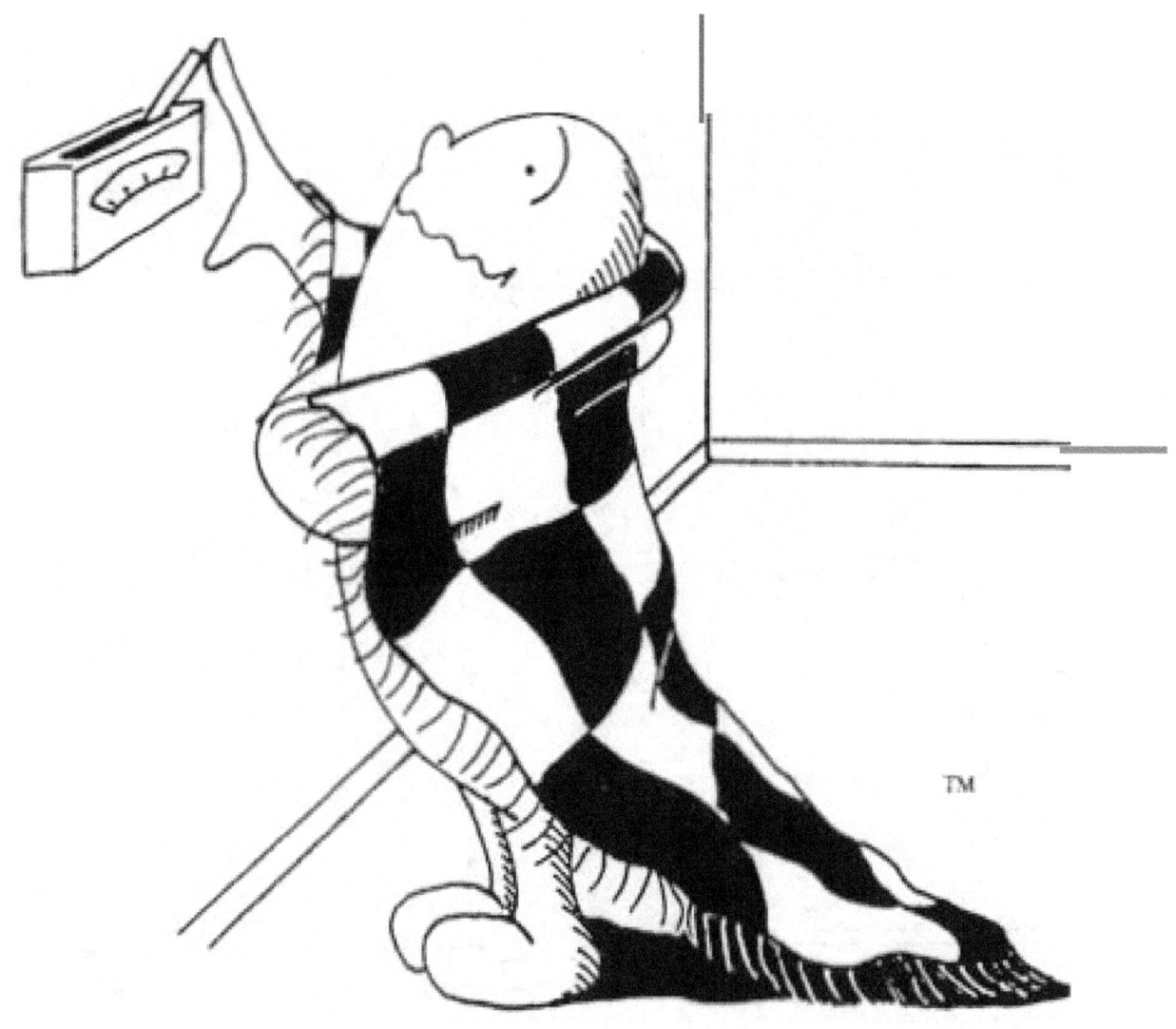

Fuel is the FOOD you eat and there are three kinds:

carbohydrates • proteins • fat

When Harmony does not get
the right fuels,
you get sick.

Fuels (food) provide nutrients for your body.

All foods should be fresh and natural.

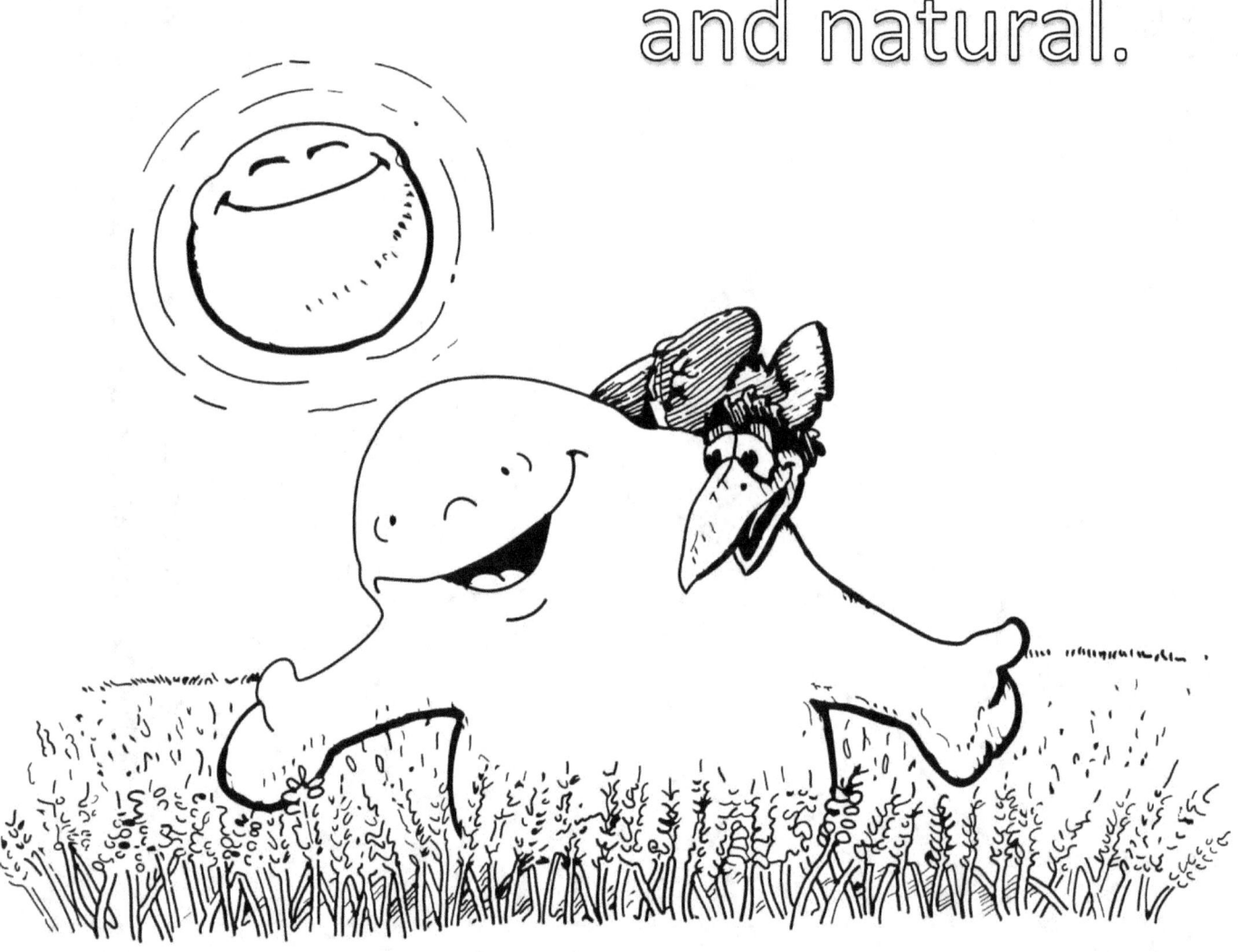

Breads made with whole grains make Harmony happy – and give you lots of energy.

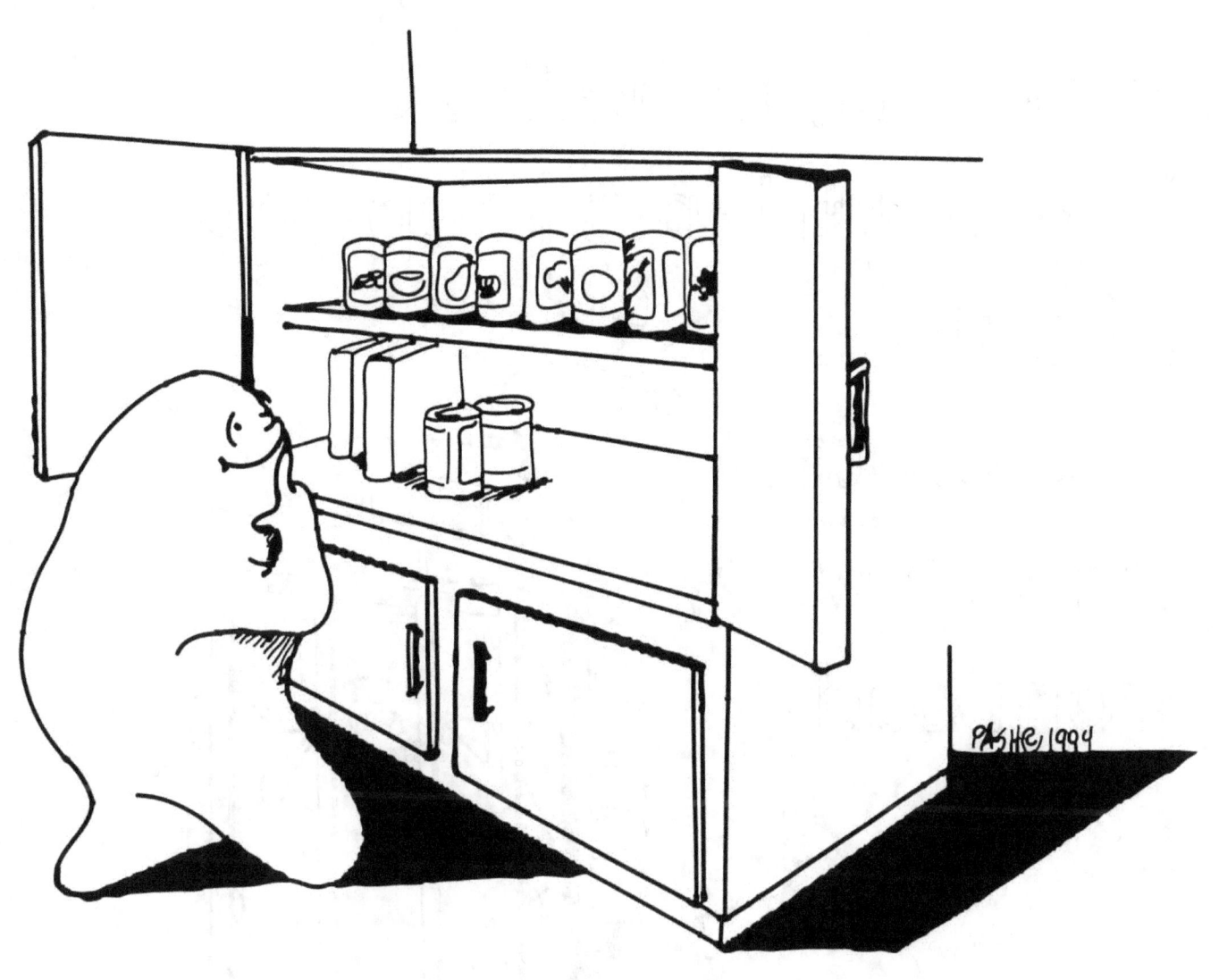

Harmony likes vitamins, minerals & phytonutrients.

Make sure your parents give you some every day.

Vitamins, minerals &
phytonutrients keep you
healthy...
and protect
Harmony
from bad
germs.

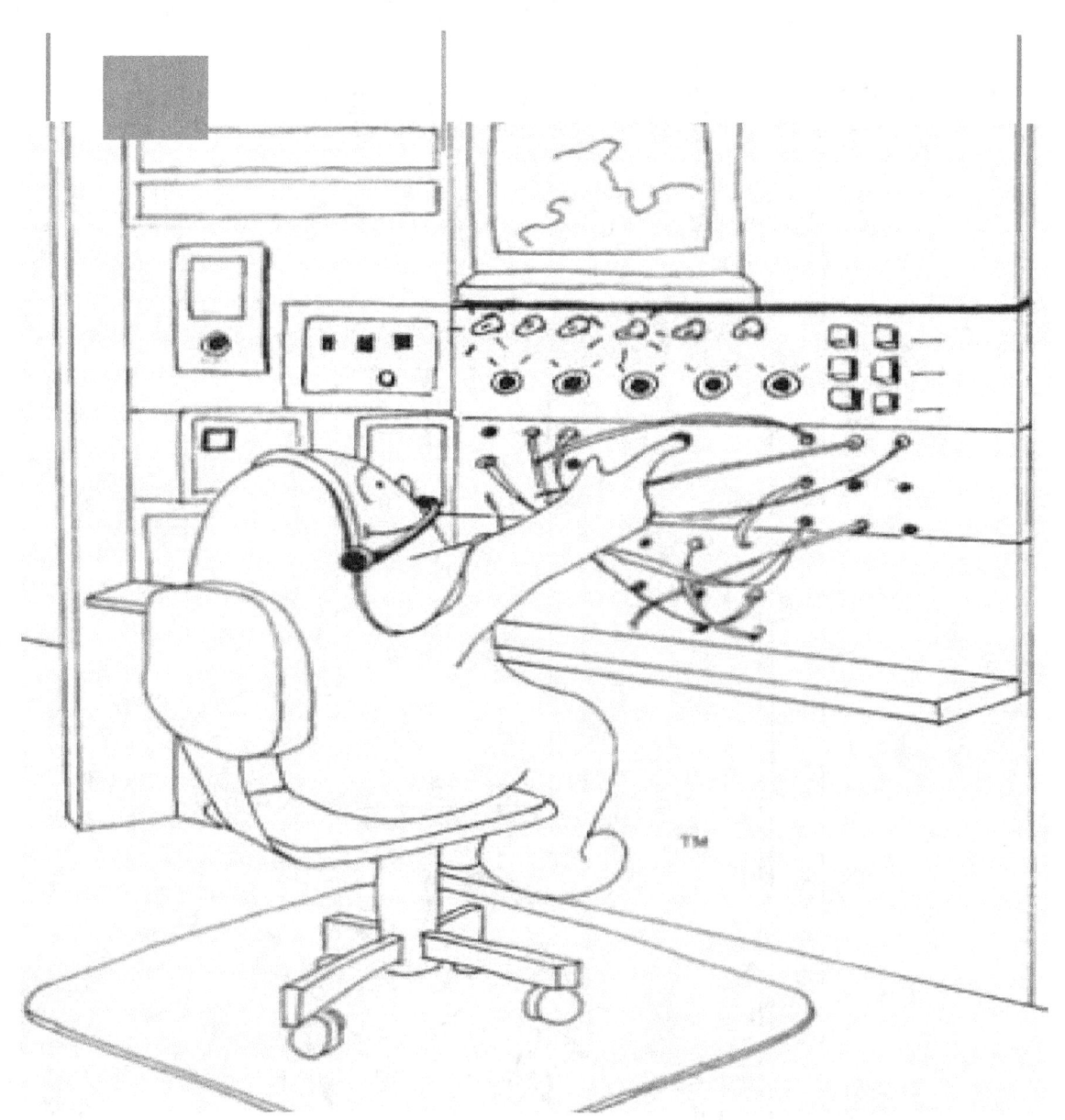

You have 100,000,000,000 brain cells that talk to all the other cells and tell them what to do. **Please don't damage your brain cells with alcohol, sugar, colas and cigarettes.**

Harmony loves exercise.
Exercise gets oxygen to all your cells.

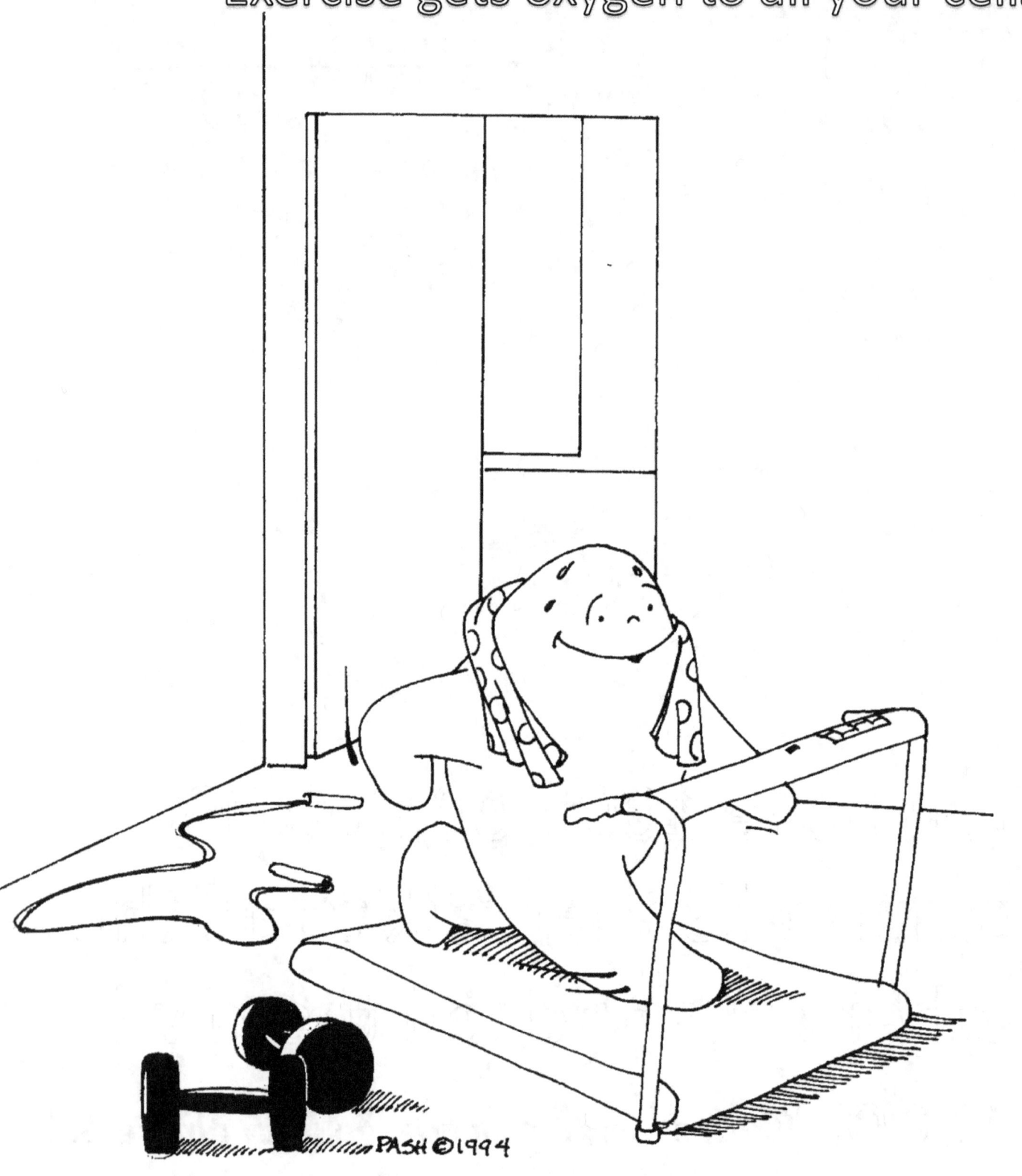

PASH ©1994

Cells need oxygen to be healthy.

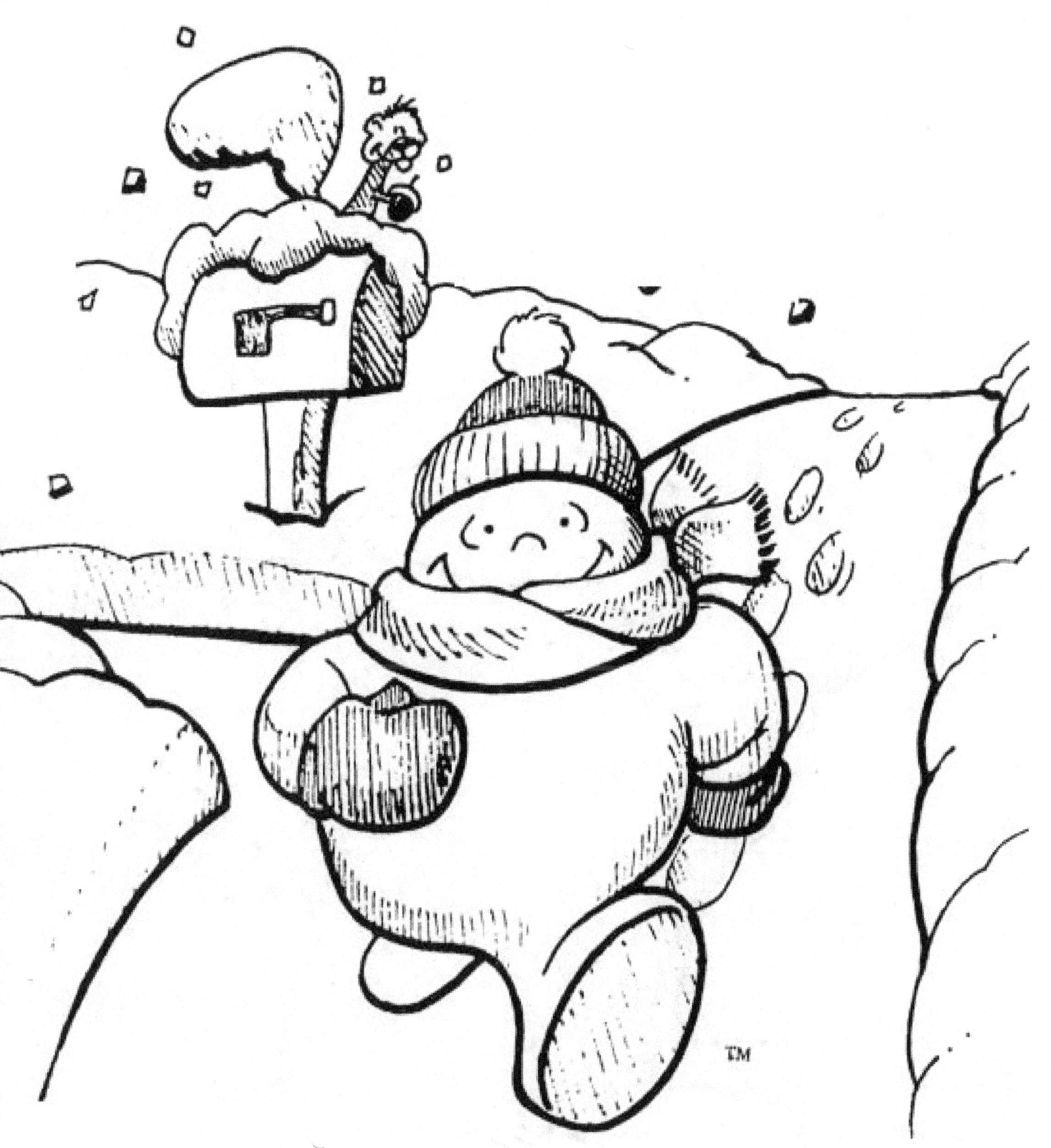

A brisk walk every day
is good exercise.

You'll feel good

& look great

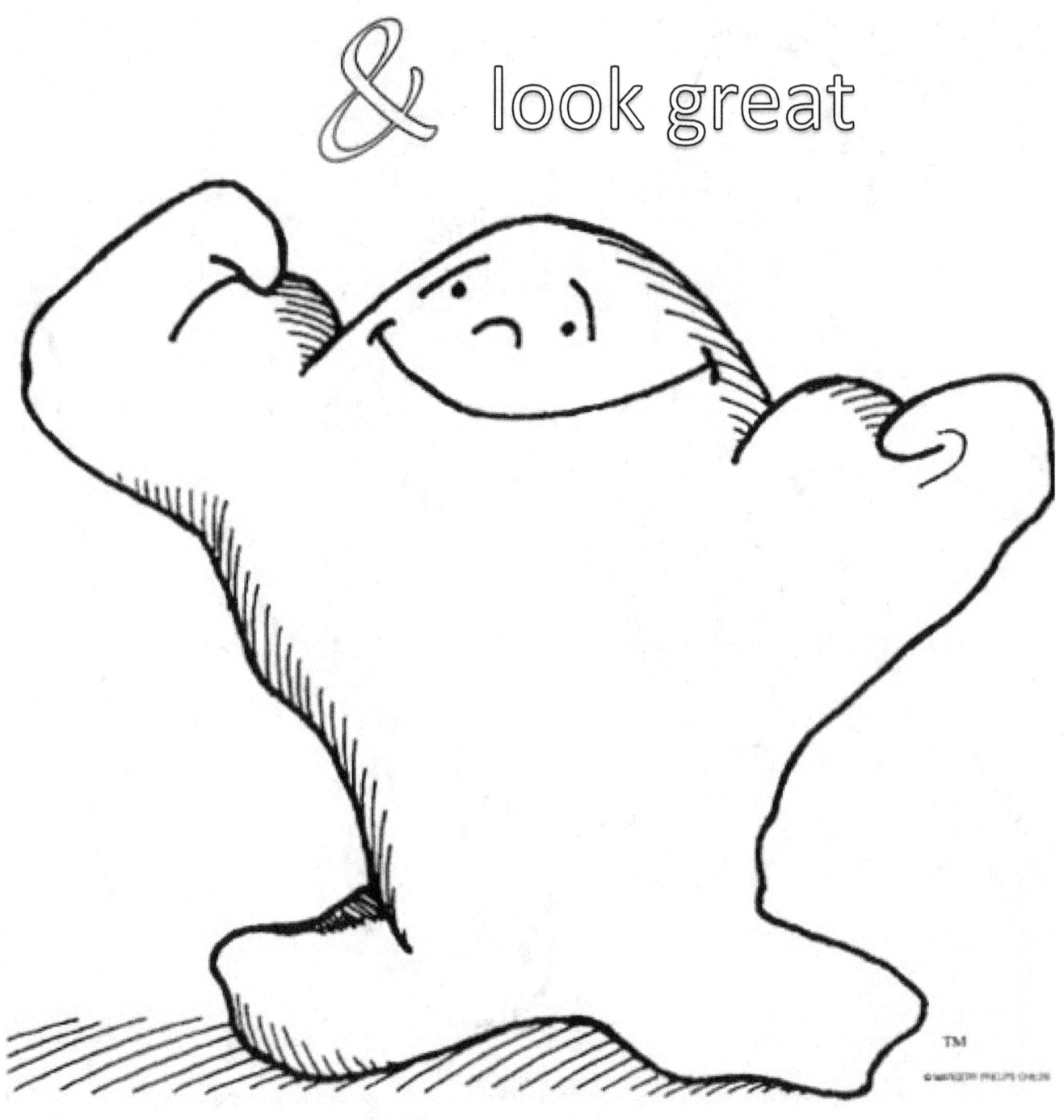

when you exercise.

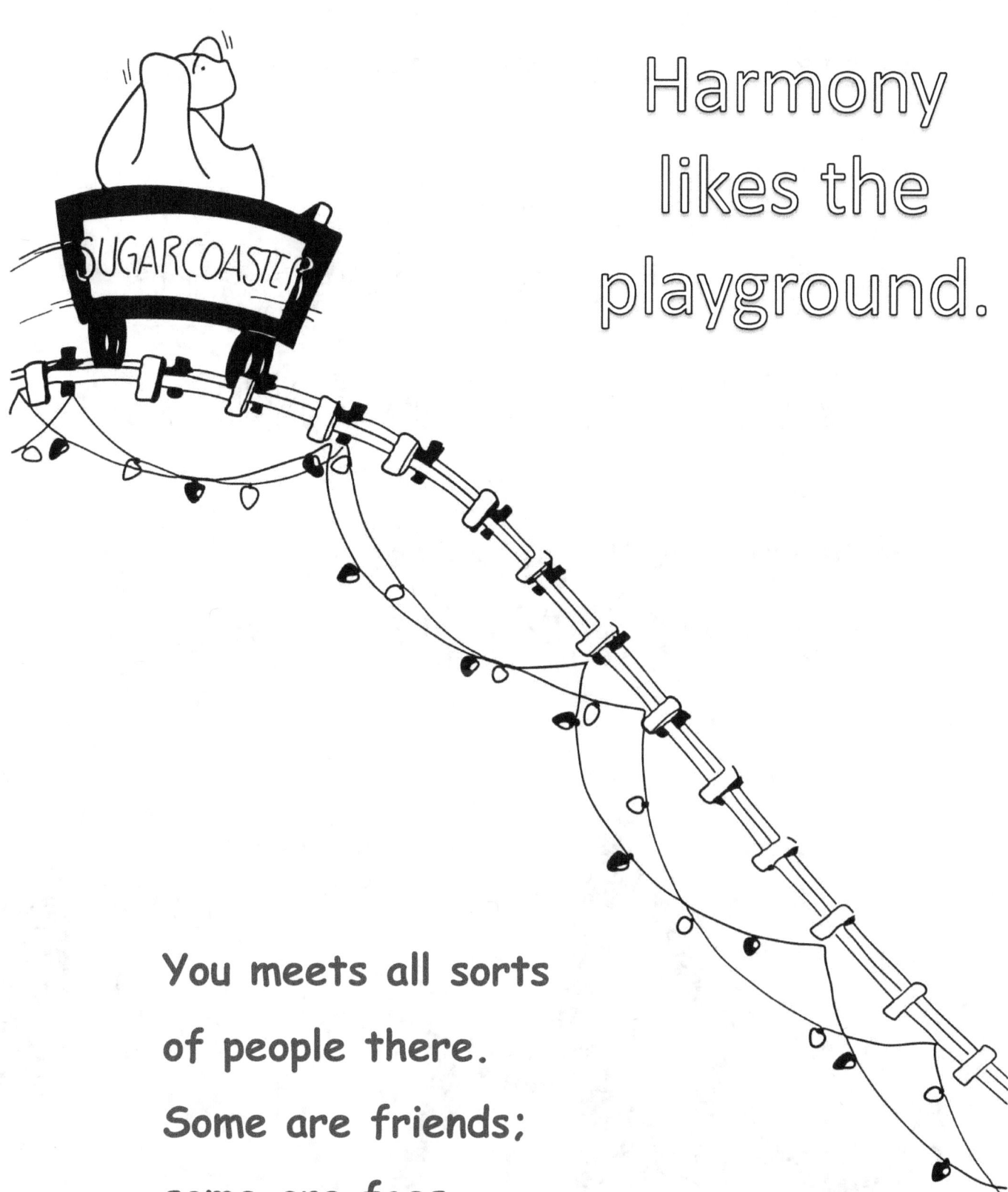

Harmony likes the playground.

You meets all sorts
of people there.
Some are friends;
some are foes.

Friends are VITAMINS & MINERALS & PHYTONUTRIENTS.

You'll crash with these foes:

Candy • Colas • Cigarettes • Drugs

So ...

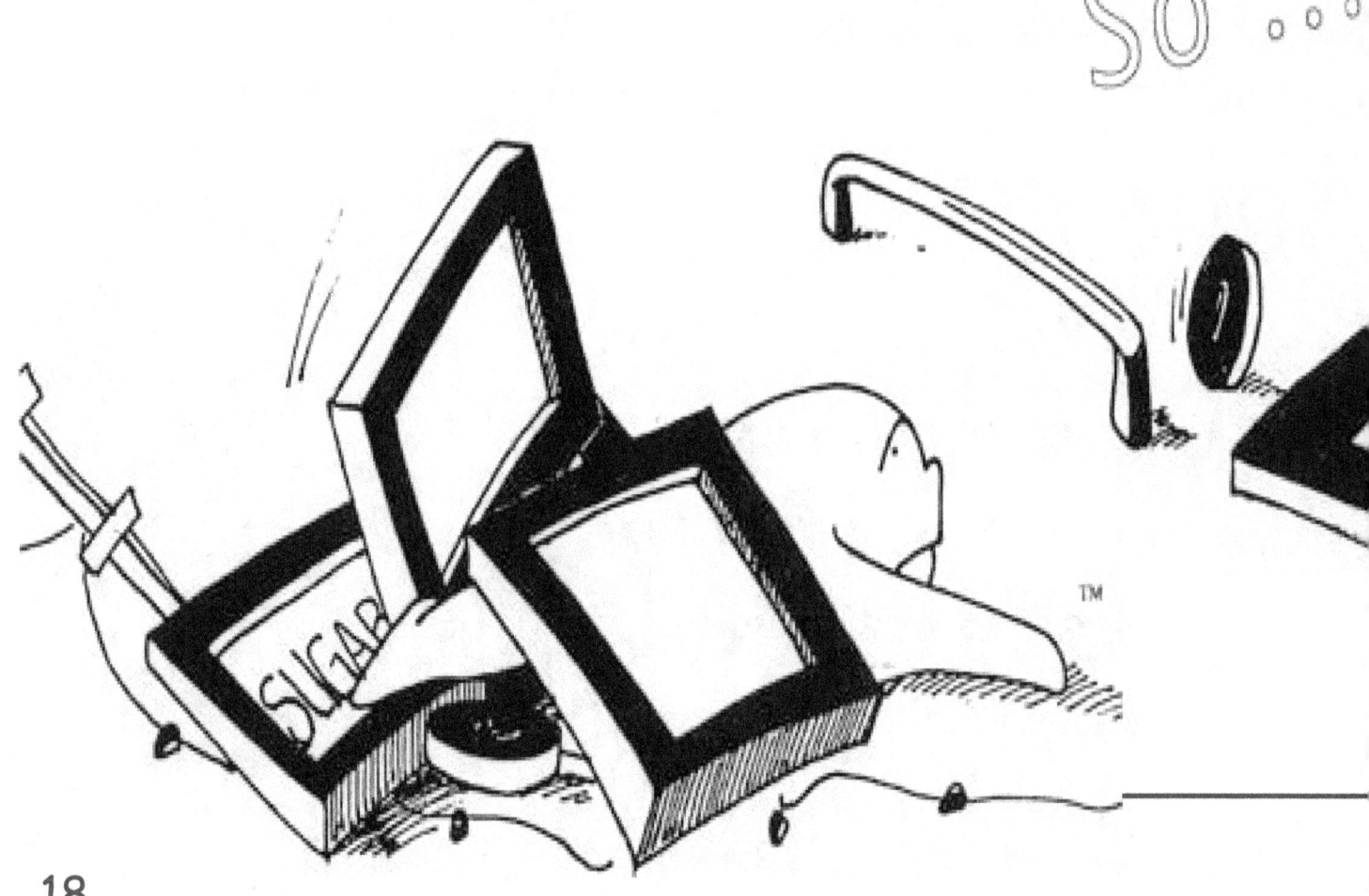

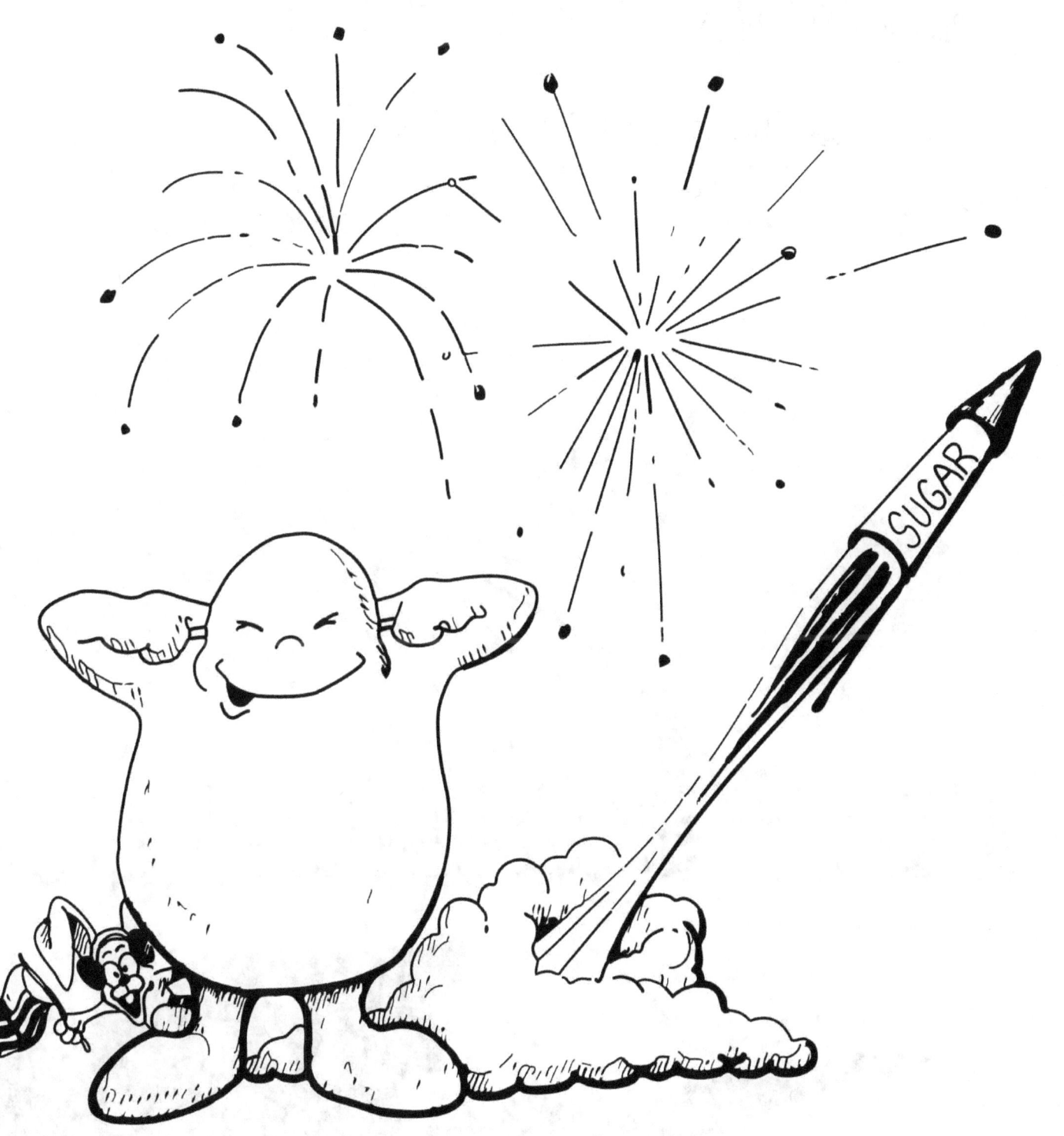

Declare your independence
from foes!

Harmony needs to relax once in a while.

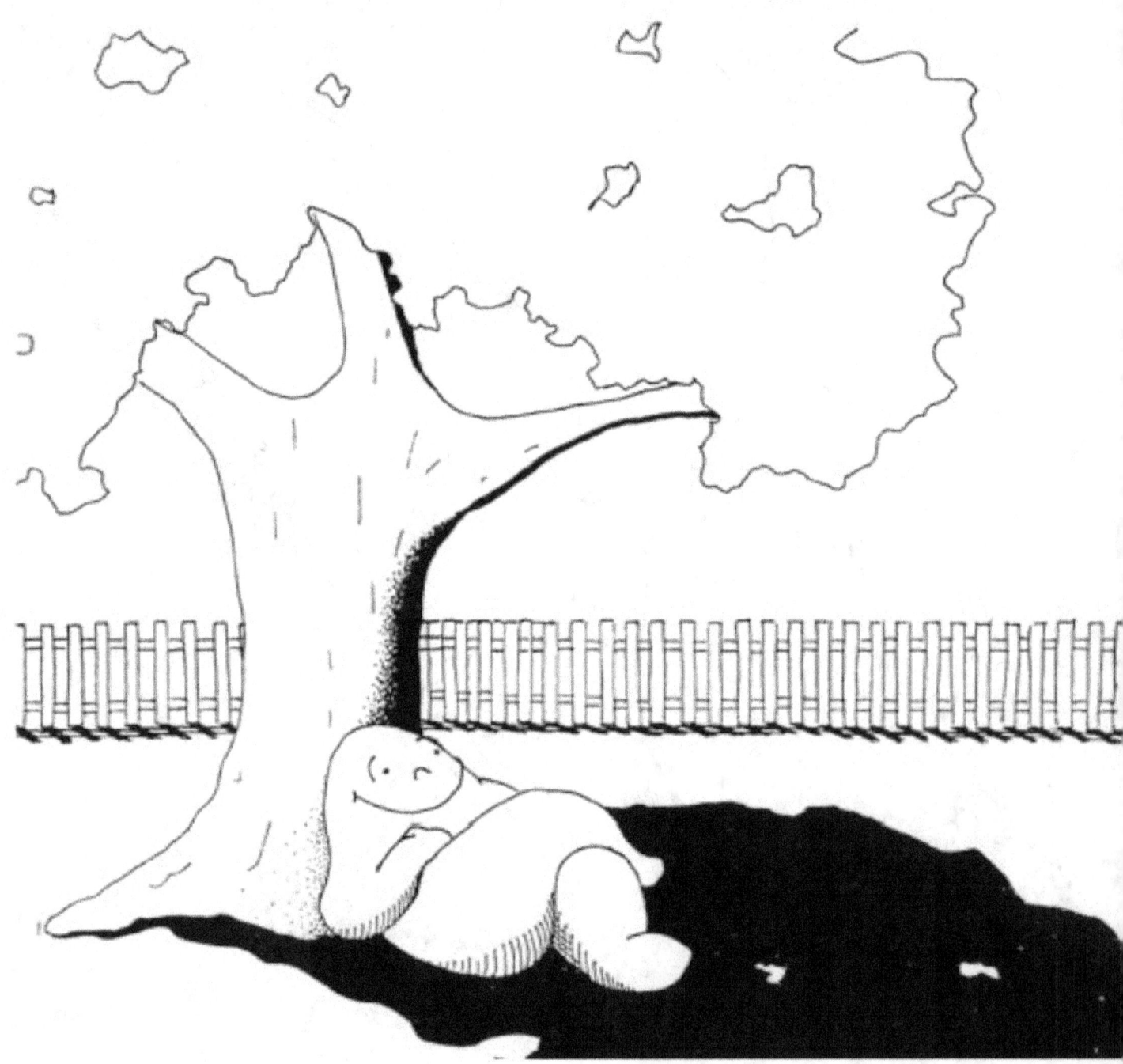

Watching TV is not relaxing.

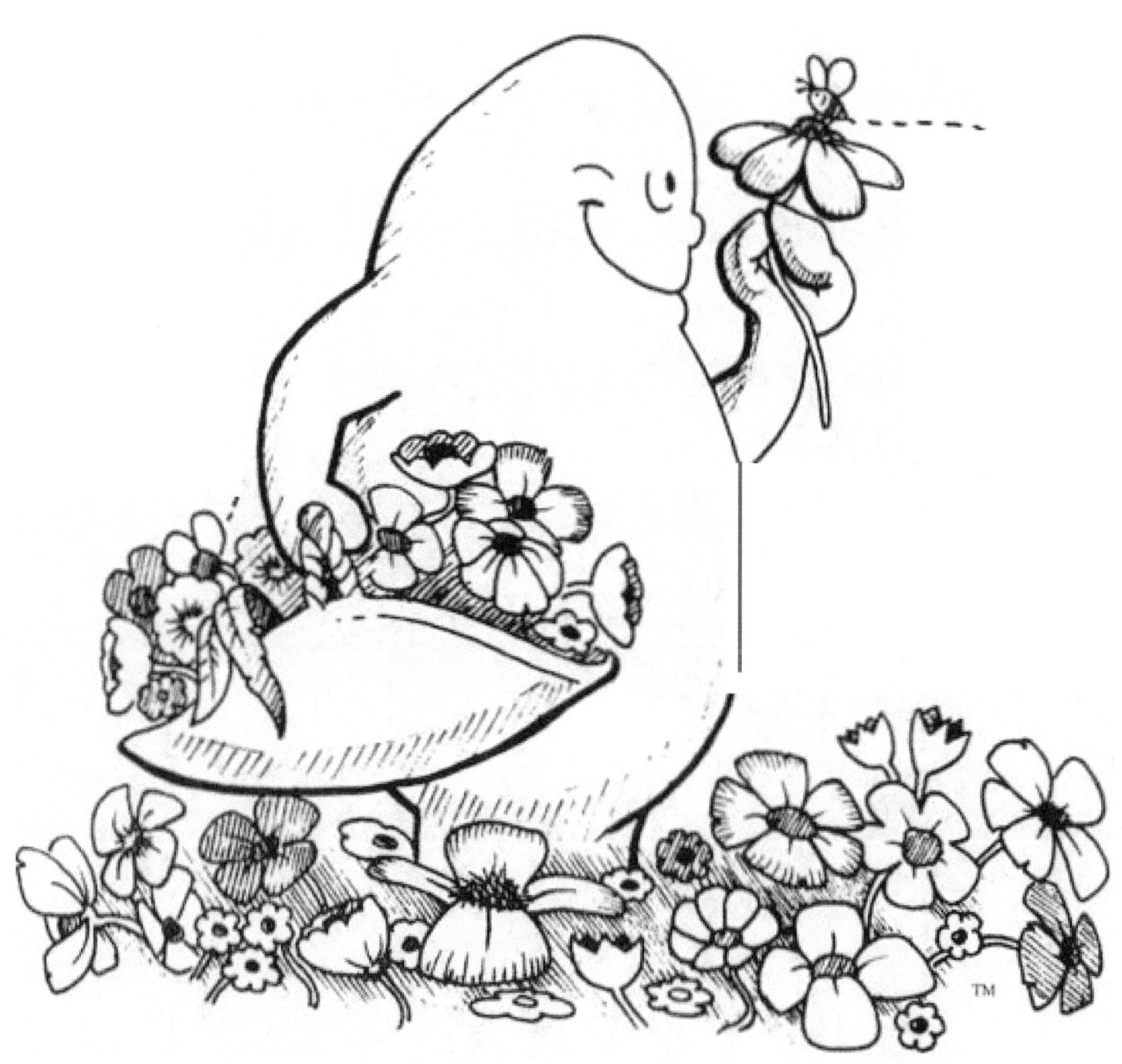

Take time to smell the flowers . . .

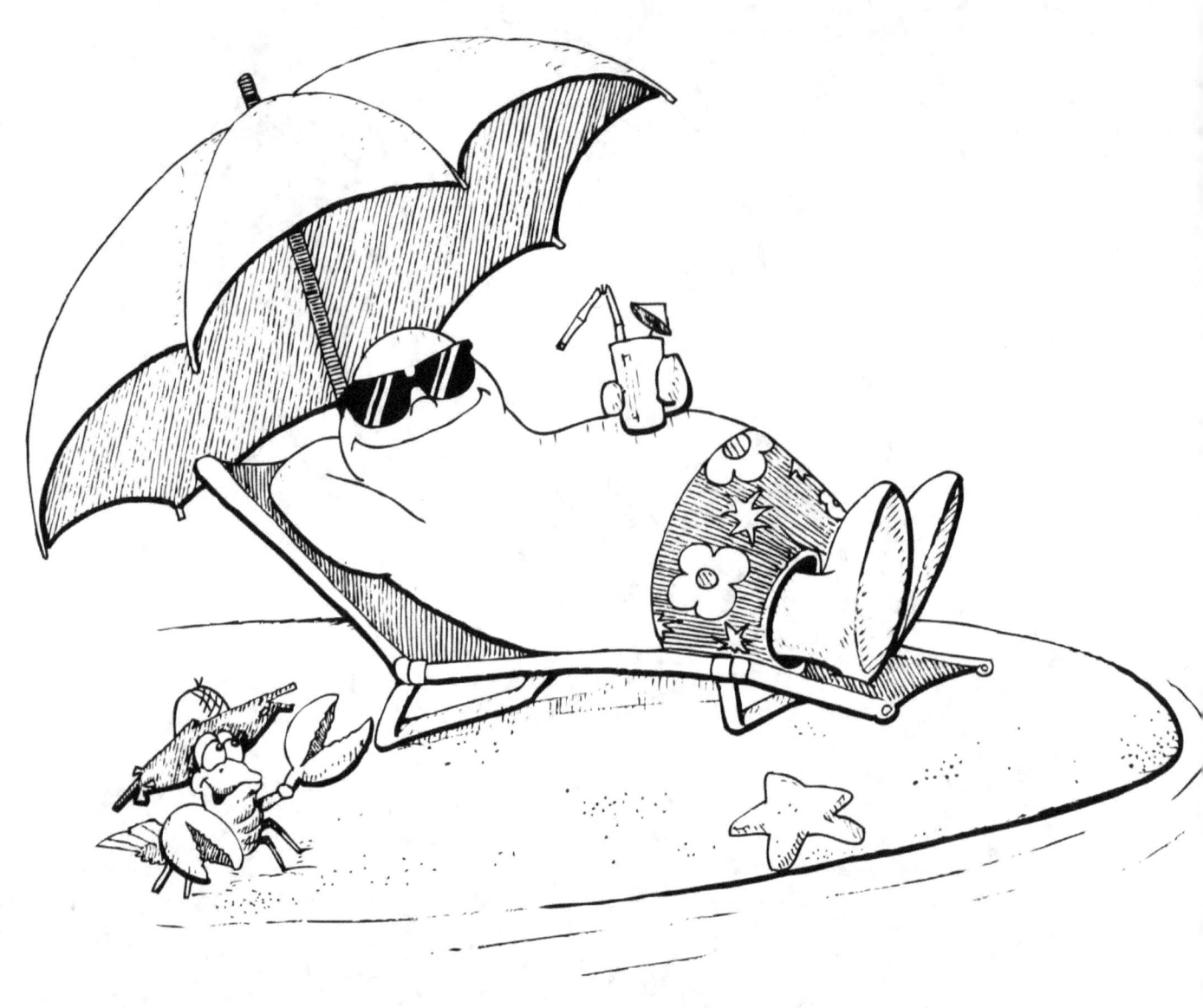

. . . and enjoy the fresh air
and sunshine.

Be sure to wear sun screen.

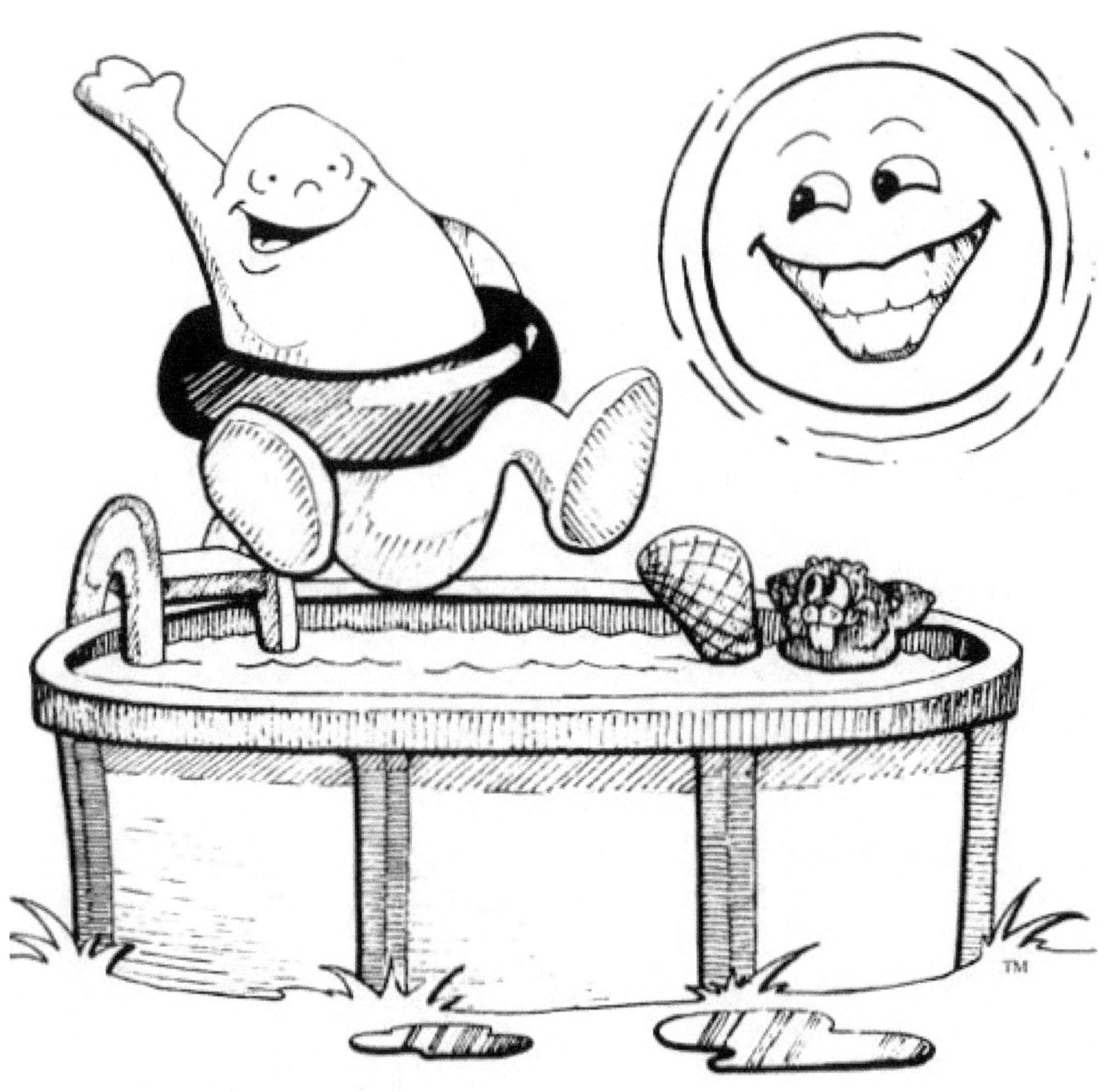

Have fun in the water . . .

don't forget your life preserver.

Pack a picnic for Harmony with fresh fruits and natural foods that have lots of good Vitamins, Minerals, and Phytonutrients . . .

And you will
Glow with Good Health
. . . Like Harmony!

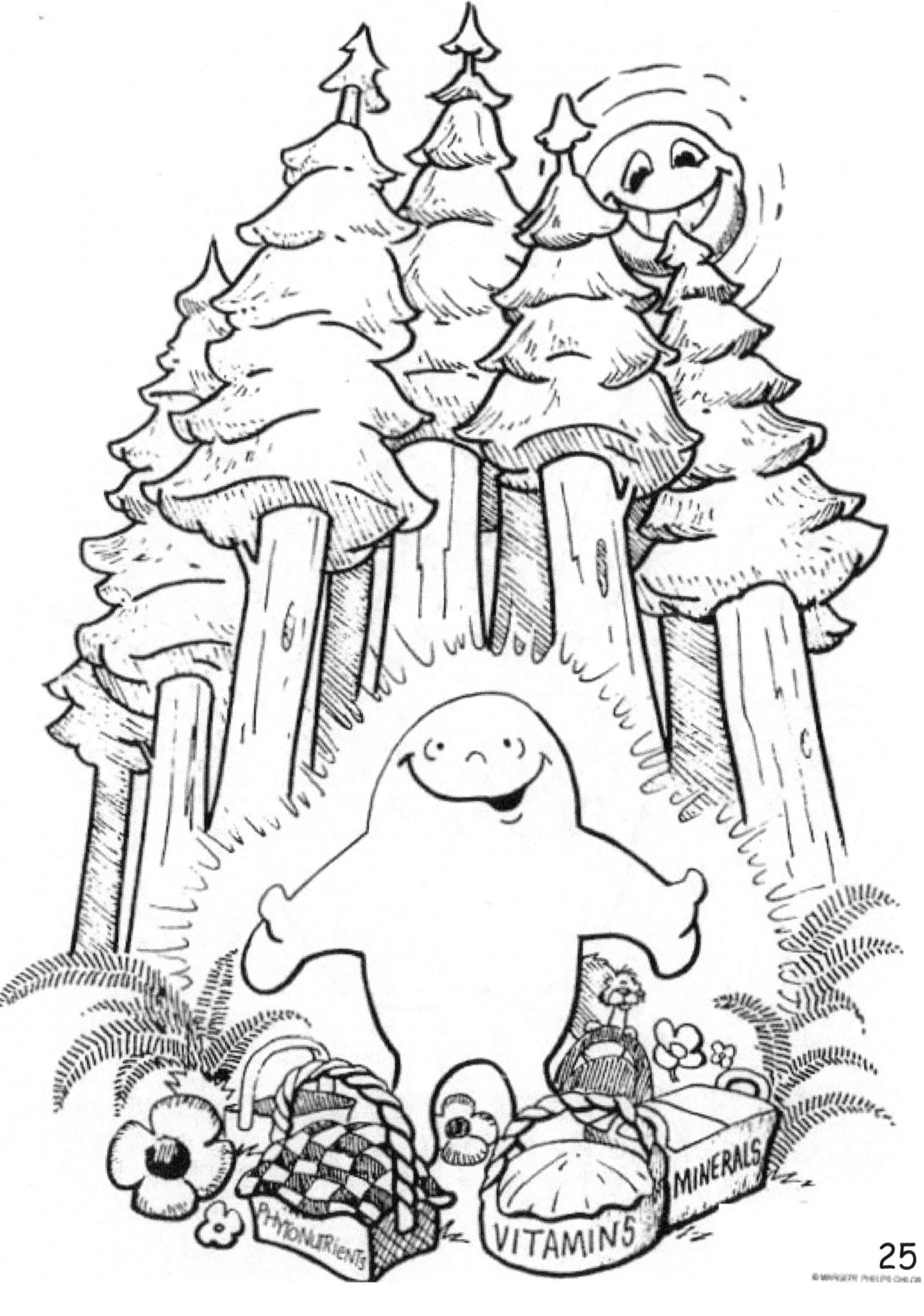

VITAMINS   MINERALS   PHYTONUTRIENTS

25

In Harmony's House we are always . . .

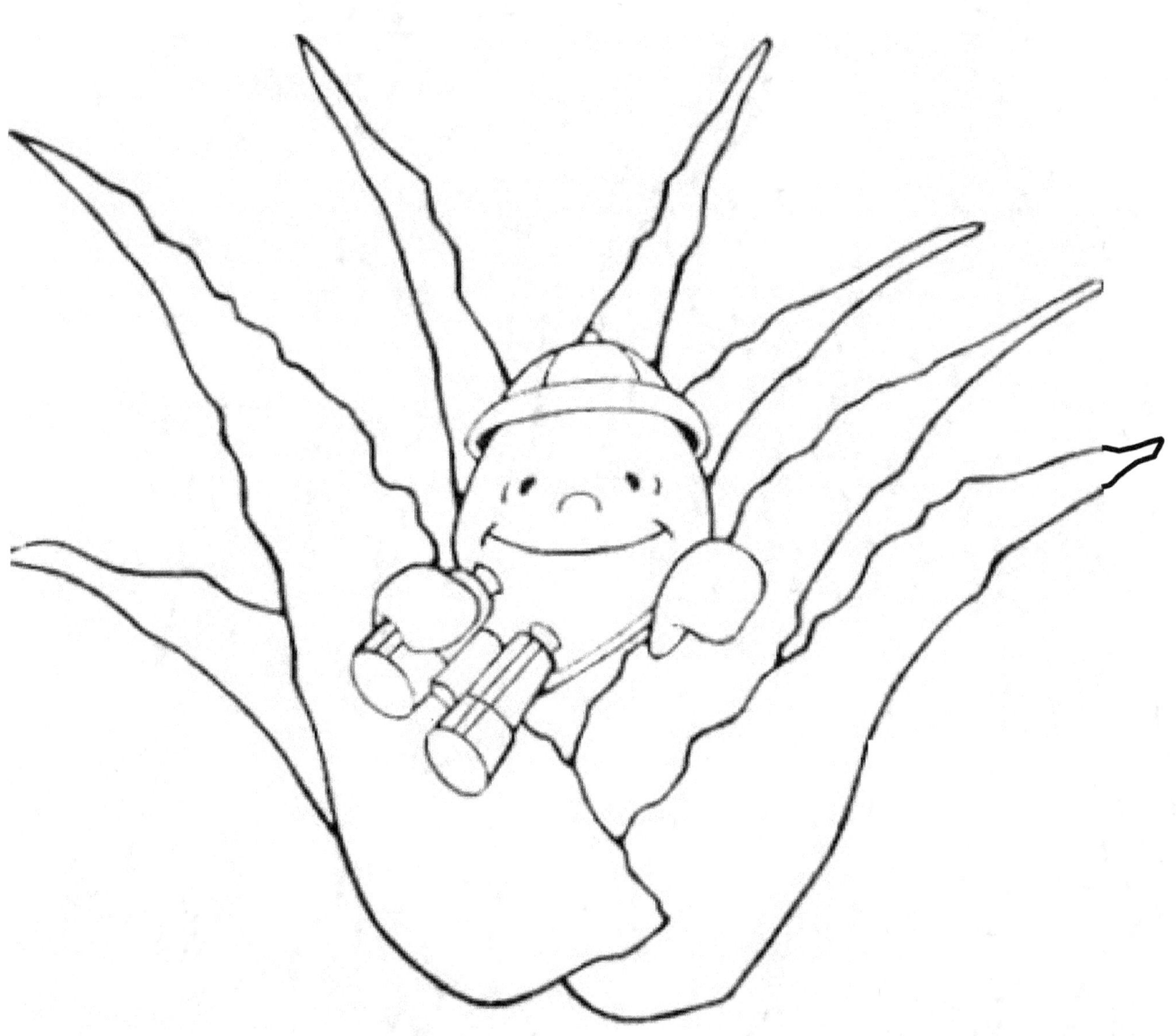

searching for Good Health.